God's Pathway to Healing

JOINTS
and
ARTHRITIS

BOOKS BY
REGINALD B. CHERRY, M.D.

―――――――

GOD'S PATHWAY TO HEALING:

Digestion

Herbs That Heal

Joints and Arthritis

Menopause

Prostate

Vision

―――――――

Dr. Cherry's Little Instruction Book

God's Pathway to Healing

JOINTS
and
ARTHRITIS

by

Reginald B. Cherry, M.D.

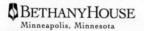
BETHANYHOUSE
Minneapolis, Minnesota

God's Pathway to Healing: Joints and Arthritis
Copyright © 2003
Reginald B. Cherry, M.D.

Page 143 is a continuation of the copyright page.

Cover design by Danielle White

Note: The directions given in this book are in no way to be considered a substitute for consultation with your own physician.

Published by Bethany House Publishers
A Ministry of Bethany Fellowship International
11400 Hampshire Avenue South
Bloomington, Minnesota 55438
www.bethanyhouse.com

Printed in the United States of America by
Bethany Press International, Bloomington, Minnesota 55438

ISBN 0-7642-2767-X

CONTENTS

INTRODUCTION: LIVING ON THE CUTTING EDGE

Arthritis is one of the most common, annoying, aggravating, and painful physical problems faced by men and women. While not often a life-threatening disease, arthritis is extremely serious because it inflicts mild to excruciating suffering upon multiplied millions of people, disturbs rest and sleep, and hinders work and normal activities.

There are more than one hundred kinds of arthritis, from the most common "worn-out-joints" osteoarthritis to rheumatoid arthritis, psoriatic arthritis, juvenile arthritis, the extremely painful gouty arthritis, Reiter's syndrome, ankylosing spondylitis—and more. Medical researchers estimate that 90 percent— nine out of ten—of those over age forty already have the beginnings of arthritis, the thinning of the cartilage in the joints. We know that osteoarthritis strikes women three times more often than men, probably for some hormone-related reason. And while long regarded as a problem of older people—70 percent of folks over sixty-five have significant symptoms— three out of five people with arthritis are *younger* than sixty-five.

This painful malady is already our leading cause of disability—even more so than heart disease and cancer! Medical statisticians predict that in the next ten years there could be as many as 110 million people partially or totally disabled by movement-limiting arthritic joints.

COUNTING THE COST OF ARTHRITIS

Arthritis is extremely expensive—not only for the seven million visits per year to doctors, soaring over-the-counter and prescription drug sales, and major surgeries, such as 250,000 total knee replacements and 150,000 artificial hip implants per year, but also in lost workdays and cancelled activities. Direct medical costs are more than $15 *billion* per year. When lost wages and other economic factors are considered, the impact on the nation is some $65 billion annually, roughly equivalent to a moderate recession, with an aggregate cost of about 1.1 percent of the gross national product.[1]

This is no minor nuisance. We're talking about a major problem that negatively impacts individuals, marriages, families, employers, churches, communities, cities, states—our entire nation.

Until very recently, medical science offered very little hope for arthritis sufferers. When I was in medical school, we were taught that arthritis was incurable. Doctors could prescribe medicines to help cope with the pain and the feverish inflammation and swelling, and that was about it. When the disease progressed to the point that joints were immobilized and patients were almost totally handicapped, then, in some cases, medical science could step in and try total knee replacement surgery or hip transplants. But these procedures didn't always bring complete relief—and the prostheses only lasted a few years. Then the surgery had to be done all over again.

IS THERE ANY GOOD NEWS?

That's the bad news! However, I have written this book to bring you words of encouragement and hope. I want you to know that God is not the author of arthritis! He doesn't want you—or any of your loved ones and friends—to suffer the pain, physical handicaps, limitations, unfulfilled plans and dreams, and financial loss of this terrible group of diseases.

His plan for you is—and always has been—good: "For I know the thoughts and plans that I have for you, says the Lord, thoughts and plans for welfare and peace and not for evil, to give you hope in your final outcome" (Jeremiah 29:11 AMP).

Well, if sickness and disease are not God's doing, where do they come from? Jesus answered this clearly during His earthly ministry when He said, "The thief comes only in order to steal and kill and destroy." If you've ever seen an arthritic patient, limbs twisted and contorted, desperately crying out from the pain and swelling, you recognize this picture. Jesus went on to say, "I came that they may have and enjoy life, and have it in abundance" (John 10:10 AMP).

Now we're talking good news! Not only did God *not* put arthritis on you and your loved ones, but He wants to take away your pain and restore your body from all the crippling symptoms. Look at this: "God anointed Jesus of Nazareth with the Holy Ghost and with power: who went about doing good, and healing all that were oppressed of the devil; for God was with him" (Acts 10:38).

With all my heart, I believe that God has a pathway to healing for your arthritis! That pathway will be uniquely yours. The Gospels relate how Jesus healed and restored sight to blind men on different occasions. He touched one and commanded him to see; He anointed others and prayed repeatedly; He put a mixture of clay and saliva on another's eyes and sent him to a pool to wash it off. The bottom line of each story is that the blind man was healed and regained his sight!

John 9:7 says the blind man "went his way therefore, and washed, and came seeing." And I tell you that as you follow *your* pathway to healing, you can be restored and made whole by the healing power of God.

Perhaps God will use conventional medicine to control your pain and the symptoms of arthritis. Maybe He will miraculously, supernaturally touch your body and make you well. It could be that you will be led to discover the healing to be found in natural substances in the form of food or supplements. Or possibly your healing will come through a combination of all these things. But there is a pathway to healing out there for you.

WHY NOT BE A PATHFINDER?

I urge you to be a pathfinder! The Bible says, "Ye have not, because ye ask not" (James 4:2). Don't make that mistake. Realize that all healing comes from God, and ask Him to heal you: "Let us then approach the throne of grace with confidence, so that we may receive mercy and find grace to help us in our time of need" (Hebrews 4:16 NIV).

There's more good news I want you to know about. Medical science is changing its mind about arthritis! By that I mean it is making a 180° change in its attitude about whether or not this disease can be cured. Where doctors once said, "There is no cure for arthritis, and sooner or later most people are going to suffer from it," a respected medical journal recently said, "But now nutritional biochemistry has changed all of this."

For more than twenty-five years my personal medical practice focused on preventive medicine—helping people stop sickness and disease before it started. The best healing, you see, is never to get an illness in the first place. As I prayed with patients and helped them seek ways to get well and stay healthy, I saw so much of God's plan in the Bible that medical science was just beginning to consider and investigate.

Several years ago medicine began to promote the use of estrogen therapy for women with reproductive disorders and other female problems. When I began to delve into the subject in my personal studies, I found that researchers had discovered more than 250 plants and substances that contained natural estrogen. From the days of creation, God had provided what was needed to protect women and their bodies.

SCIENCE IS PLAYING CATCH-UP

This is why I so often say that science is always playing catch-up, walking in the footsteps of God. Now we're finding the same thing is true about arthritis. More and more of the influential medical journals are telling us doctors that we are no longer limited to easing the pain of arthritis and trying to alleviate the effects of inflammation in the joints. Now we can do something to *prevent* the development of painful symptoms—and to *restore* worn and damaged cartilage in the joints.

No, it's not yet a total cure—but it's definitely the first steps on that road! I've been personally researching this whole field for months. I've enlisted the services of a skilled team of medical researchers—Ph.D.s in chemistry, and other physicians—to search out what natural substances and compounds are available to combat arthritis and carve out a pathway to healing and restoration.

I'm so excited to be living on the cutting edge, on the forefront of where medical science is going. I believe we are seeing the various healing streams starting to flow together to bless all of humankind.

In this book I want to share with you the information you need to find help for your own body or for your loved ones. Even if you've been disappointed in the past, or you've failed to do your part to live in health, it's not too late. There is still hope and healing for you.

You will need to be "doers of the word, and not hearers only, deceiving your own selves" (James 1:22). God has entrusted you with the responsibility of protecting and caring for your "temple." Let's get started on your pathway to healing.

"He that hath ears to hear, let him hear" (Matthew 11:15).

Chapter 1

THERE IS SOMETHING YOU CAN DO ABOUT ARTHRITIS

Chapter 1

THERE IS SOMETHING YOU CAN DO ABOUT ARTHRITIS

As I've pointed out, our understanding of arthritis has changed dramatically in the past few years. While on the one hand it threatens to be our next epidemic and is still a major cause of disability, medical researchers are now changing their minds about arthritis being incurable.

A quote in a recent medical journal stated that "until very recently arthritis was incurable, part of old age—and we are all eventually going to succumb, *but now nutritional biochemistry has changed all this*" (emphasis mine). In short, now there is something we can do about arthritis besides accepting and enduring it.

As a Christian physician, from a biblical point of view, I believe that arthritis is a formidable attack against humankind, designed not only to cause us inconvenience and painful discomfort but ultimately to immobilize us and cripple us. In fact, it has become the leading cause of disability.

Arthritis comes in over one hundred different forms and affects 43 million Americans—one in every six. The truth is that if we remain passive about arthritis, it is going to increase dramatically. Estimates indicate that it will affect anywhere from 40 to 100 million people by the year 2020.

Studies show that 90 percent of people

over the age of forty already have the beginning stages of arthritis. If you are twenty pounds overweight, you are likely to have osteoarthritis in your joints. Seventy percent of people over the age of sixty-five have joint symptoms related to arthritis.

DIFFERENT RESULTS REQUIRE DIFFERENT METHODS

Traditional medicine uses pain-killers and anti-inflammatories, including a new class of drugs known as COX–2 inhibitors (Celebrex and Vioxx). COX–2 refers to the enzyme *cyclooxygenase–2*, which triggers the production of inflammation and pain in arthritic joints. By inhibiting, or restraining, the development of inflammation or swelling, these expensive prescription-only drugs are very effective in relieving discomfort, although they have potentially serious drawbacks when synthesized in a laboratory. They appear to be linked to increased incidence of kidney problems and heart disease.

Amazingly, God made a different form of COX–2 inhibitors—readily available to us in the plant kingdom—that do not have these distressing side effects. We will discuss these in detail a little later. In addition, there are ways to prevent arthritis. If you already have been diagnosed with it, there are ways to reverse the course of the disease.

First, some background on arthritis. Researchers now know that osteoarthritis (the most common type, which we will focus on primarily) results from a wearing down of cartilage on the surface of bones. Cartilage is an amazing substance consisting of approximately

90 percent water and having almost no friction.

Pushing an ice cube across a wet kitchen counter will send it flying. Cartilage is twice as slippery. Another amazing fact is that it is one of the few areas in the body that has no blood supply. It receives all its nutrients by circulation through its fluids.

What causes arthritis?

The cause of arthritis is difficult to define. Most researchers now feel that, contrary to popular opinion, it is not a normal part of aging, with cartilage simply wearing out from use over time. They point out that patients use both of their knees at the same rate, but arthritis frequently attacks only one knee.

Again, women are three times more likely to suffer from osteoarthritis than men, presumably because of hormonal activity. This is why the use of soy, isoflavones, and other flavonoid compounds may be particularly helpful to women, in addition to protecting them from hot flashes and osteoporosis, which is actual bone loss.

While obesity is suspected to be a major risk factor for osteoarthritis of the knees and hips because of the increased load on these weight-bearing joints, it has not yet been absolutely proven. A more conclusive risk factor appears to be previous trauma or joint injury, often from sports or work-related mishaps. Knee injuries that seemingly heal well—even those that occur in the teen years—may actually set the stage for future arthritis.

In fact, one study indicated that teenagers who incurred a knee injury were three times more likely to experience arthritis in later years. Even torn or stretched ligaments around the knees and hips can contribute to arthritis by leading to instability in the joint.

FROM ONE EXTREME TO THE OTHER

Traditional medicine has typically treated arthritis in two extremes. First, with a class of drugs known as NSAIDs (for "nonsteroidal anti-inflammatory drugs"), such as aspirin, ibuprofen (Advil, Nuprin), and naproxen sodium (Aleve), and more recently, with the COX-2 inhibitors (Celebrex and Vioxx), all of which work pretty well at relieving the pain. Second, at the other extreme, by removing the affected joint and replacing it with a prosthesis, or artificial joint. Surgeons are now performing more than 250,000 total knee replacements annually and more than 150,000 artificial hip implants.

The downside to NSAIDs is that about 25

percent of the patients who used them for an extended period of time experienced indigestion, nausea, vomiting, peptic ulcers, and damage to the kidneys. The COX–2 inhibitors, besides costing as much as $3 per pill, tend to increase kidney and heart disease. Joint replacement provides remarkable relief for many, but the life expectancy of the artificial joint averages only ten to fifteen years; then it has to be replaced in another surgery.

Is there any form of treatment in between? Does God have a pathway for healing using natural means? Medical research increasingly indicates that natural compounds are indeed proving not only to treat the pain and inflammation of arthritis but also to possibly restore cartilage itself—something medicine cannot do except with artificial joints.

With the existing and projected numbers

of arthritis sufferers, it is obvious that what is needed is not only a treatment plan but an effective preventive plan as well. Our goal should be wholeness, not simply symptom control.

GOD'S 3–2–3 PLAN

Three categories must be addressed in dealing with arthritis: pain, inflammation, and restoration of cartilage. God has provided three natural substances to deal with pain, two to decrease inflammation, and three to actually restore cartilage. I call this God's 3–2–3 approach to joint health. Let's look at these categories one by one.

First, God's plan does not include painful cartilage deterioration resulting from arthritis until standing or walking causes bone to grind against bone. In fact, God has provided the same COX–2 inhibitors for relieving pain (as well as inflammation) that expensive prescription drugs relieve—without the side effects. These natural COX–2 inhibitors restrain a class of hormones known as *prostaglandins,* but they have no ill effects on the stomach.

Many of nature's compounds contain small amounts of COX–2 inhibitors, but three in particular stand out. Let's get your pain stopped and then work on restoring your cartilage.

The first compound is actually a cousin to ginger and has a yellowish pigment called *curcumin* derived from the curcuma root. It is also known as turmeric root, and you may recognize this as the compound that is found in curry powder. Curcumin, or curcuma root, has been used for centuries as a pain-killer and anti-inflammatory.

If it weren't effective, it would have long since been abandoned, but over the centuries people kept turning to curcuma for relief of their symptoms. They weren't chemists. They didn't know it was a COX–2 inhibitor, and they didn't call it by the name that scientists use today (a "non-steroidal anti-inflammatory drug"). They just knew it worked, so they kept using it.

Recognizing its long history of usage, medical researchers began studying this compound. Scientists at Cornell University began wondering what was in curcuma root that made it work. They discovered that, in fact, it was a COX–2 inhibitor, just like Celebrex or Vioxx, but without the side effects or price tag. They even discovered how it worked. A daily dosage of 100 mg. of curcuma root inhibited prostaglandin E2 and decreased inflammation and joint pain very effectively.

Recent breaking news about ongoing research on laboratory-produced COX–2 inhibitors indicates that they may also decrease colon cancer, which suggests that the natural plant compounds that are COX–2 inhibitors also likely offer protective benefits against this common cancer.

COULD YOU EAT TWENTY TART CHERRIES A DAY?

The next natural compound that helps stop arthritis pain is found in tart cherries—the same ones used to make cherry pie. If you've ever tried eating one of these tart cherries, you know that they are *really sour*. I mean, they will make your mouth pucker—and then you've got to spit out the pit.

Tart cherries have also been used for centuries to treat arthritis and gout. Once again, scientists noted this long-standing usage and decided to do research on it, this time at Michigan State University. Using modern laboratory testing techniques, they discovered that extracts from tart cherries also had COX–2 inhibitors, as well as compounds such as *ursolic* and *oleonolic acids*, which are ten times more active and effective than aspirin.

To quote the scientists:

> We found some powerful natural anti-inflammatory compounds that had no side effects. The cherries contain chemicals called anthocyanins, which give the red color and also seem to have an effect on inflammation. Considered

antioxidants, which neutralize agents called free radicals that cause cell damage, anthocyanins also appear to offer protection against certain cancers and cardiovascular diseases.[1]

To get the needed amount of COX–2 inhibitors to fight the pain of arthritis, you would have to eat twenty raw tart cherries a day—that's a lot of puckering and spitting! Fortunately, God has given us the wisdom to extract the beneficial compounds from the cherries and make it available in tart cherry powder (I recommend about 100 mg. a day). I promise you it is a lot easier on the taste buds!

HOLY BASIL—WHAT'S THAT STUFF?

No, it's not the same as the common herb basil, but the healing qualities of holy basil have been recognized for five thousand years in its native India. Like curcumin and tart cherries, this herb also has chemical compounds containing natural COX–2 inhibitors with anti-inflammatory effectiveness similar to aspirin and ibuprofen. Unlike the NSAIDs, holy basil is not irritating to the stomach and, in fact, has properties that help to prevent ulcers caused by these drugs. A dose of 150 mg. daily is recommended in combination with curcumin and tart cherry powder.

Now that we have dealt with the pain, let's get closer to the source of the problem by dealing with the inflammation that actually causes the redness, swelling, stiffness, and ultimately the pain in the joints. There are two interesting natural compounds in this category—the middle section of God's 3–2–3 approach to joint health.

THE HEALING QUALITY OF FRANKINCENSE

In the gospel of Matthew's account of the Christmas story, we learn that wise men, or magi, from the East visited the baby Jesus and presented treasured gifts of gold, frankincense, and myrrh. Until recently, I wasn't aware that frankincense, a prized fragrance, is a gum resin from the boswellia tree that is frequently used as an anti-inflammatory compound.

Carpenters and other workers of Jesus' time often rubbed frankincense on their hands and joints to reduce swelling and to relieve the pain of inflammation. It worked! No wonder it was a treasure!

Because of the clear record of ancient usage, frankincense (or boswellin) captured the attention of science. In analyzing this gum resin, a potent anti-inflammatory compound called *boswellic acid* was discovered. While effective when applied topically—rubbing it on the outside—it also worked when concentrated in a capsule and taken by mouth.

A controlled study of 150 people suffering the symptoms of arthritis produced these astounding results from using boswellic acid: 70 percent got complete relief from morning joint stiffness, and 97 percent reported "some level" of improvement. Amazing!

Scientists were so intrigued that they continued to study boswellic acid and found that it blocked the common chemical compound *leukotrienes* in the body. This has now been identified as the substance that leads to inflammation, decreased joint mobility, and misshapen and deformed joints. Boswellin can now be taken daily at a dosage of 200 mg. to obtain relief from the arthritic symptom of inflammation.

THIS IS NO PICKLE!

Another interesting compound that blocks inflammation comes from the sea cucumber, also known as *Beche-de-Mer*. This is not a plant but a marine animal related to starfish and sea urchins. This compound has been used in China for thousands of years as a treatment for arthritis.

Modern research has confirmed that substances found in sea cucumbers are beneficial for musculoskeletal inflammatory diseases, especially osteoarthritis, rheumatoid arthritis, and ankylosing spondylitis, a rheumatic disease that affects the spine. Researchers believe that sea cucumbers improve the balance of prostaglandins, which regulate the inflammatory process. They also contain various vitamins and minerals, as well as substances known as *muco-polysaccharides* and *chondroitins*, often lacking in people with arthritis and connective tissue disorders.[2]

Sea cucumbers are harvested from the sea, dried, and pulverized into powder. A dosage of 100 mg. daily in capsule form decreases redness and joint swelling by blocking *macro-phages, neutrophils,* and *monocytes,* blood cells involved in the buildup of inflammation. This is an effective compound to use with the boswellin from frankincense.

We have now seen two major ways God has given us to attack arthritis—compounds that relieve pain and compounds that relieve inflammation. The third part of God's 3–2–3 plan is actual restoration of the damaged cartilage. This restoration and reversal of cartilage destruction is truly exciting to scientists. For the first time, medicine, through natural compounds, may be able to do more than merely treat symptoms, and it provides an alternative to waiting until the arthritic damage has progressed until there is nothing left to do but resort to radical joint-replacement surgery.

GETTING TO THE ROOT OF THE PROBLEM

The breakthrough study of the natural substance *glucosamine* was reported in a recent article in the prestigious medical journal *Lancet*. Two hundred and twelve people participated in the study. Half took glucosamine, a natural substance derived from the shells of certain deep-sea animals. The other half took a placebo, or sugar pill.

The study went on not only for a few weeks or months but for three years. At the end of thirty-six months the results were amazing. Those on 1,500 mg. of glucosamine per day had a 25 percent improvement in joint symptoms. The symptoms of those on the placebo (the inactive pill) actually got worse. But it gets even better!

Those on glucosamine lost an incredible 80 percent less cartilage than those taking the dummy pill. For the first time, scientists have hinted that we may have a preventive compound available. Not only are we stopping the pain and inflammation, but with God's help we are also getting to the root of the problem and stopping the loss of cartilage.

The prevention of pain with the natural compounds noted above takes place rather quickly, but the effects of the glucosamine (which also relieves pain) can take up to two or three months. I recommend a combination of glucosamine hydrochloride and glucosamine sulfate for a combination of 1,500 mg. daily. The sulfate has been studied somewhat more, but the HCL, or hydrochloride component, may be even better. Therefore, a combination seems to be the way to go.

A NEW ERA FOR ARTHRITIS TREATMENT

The School of Public Health at the University of California has dared to pose an interesting question: "Are we entering a new era for the treatment of arthritis?" For the first time, X rays have demonstrated that arthritis can literally be stopped! Cartilage loss can actually cease.

Medicine's approach to stopping pain is laudable. No one wants to be in pain. But what good does it do to simply stop pain if the cartilage continues to deteriorate and you eventually wind up needing the radical joint replacement procedure?

Fortunately, studies like the *Lancet* study are prompting scientists to examine in depth natural compounds rather than just synthetic, laboratory-created chemicals. As they look at glucosamine, they are finding the exact mechanism for stopping cartilage deterioration. It produces compounds known as *proteoglycans,* complex hydrophilic (literally, "water-loving") compounds that help maintain the thick cushion in cartilage by attracting water. Remember—cartilage is 90 percent water.

One comment about glucosamine—it does not appear to have any side effects, including any adverse effect on diabetes. Earlier concerns that it may increase blood-sugar levels have proven to be unfounded.

We are beginning to see an unfolding pattern here. Instead of using one or two particular compounds, we find the best approach is to use multiple compounds in combination—the same way God supplies multiple chemical compounds to us when we eat a variety of foods.

Combining natural pain-killers such as curcumin and tart cherries with anti-inflammatories such as boswellin and cartilage restorers such as glucosamine, we are really seeing a multi-pronged ability to attack the curse of arthritis. Another compound that works best when combined with glucosamine and other anti-inflammatories is *chondroitin*.

ANOTHER BREAKTHROUGH!

We have actually had a breakthrough in chondroitin and overcome a problem that has challenged scientists for many years. Chondroitin traditionally has been very difficult to absorb into the body because of its high molecular weight. Dosages as high as 1,200 mg. were used, but the high molecular weight kept it from being absorbed.

We now have discovered a low-molecular-weight chondroitin that is absorbed much better at a dosage of only 100 mg. For those with a scientific background, the traditional chondroitin was approximately 18,000 daltons, which is a measure of the molecular weight. The new compound is approximately 9,000 daltons. This translates to a higher absorption at a lower dosage.

Why is chondroitin important in joint health? It is technically a *glycosaminoglycan* that holds water in the cartilage and keeps it elastic. This, in turn, allows molecules to circulate freely throughout the cartilage (remember, cartilage has no blood vessels).

I would not recommend using chondroitin by itself, as almost every study I have reviewed indicates it works best when combined with other compounds—especially glucosamine. These compounds are so promising that the National Institute of Health (NIH) is spending $14 million to study them over a long-term period (the results won't be available until 2005).

Believe me, the NIH does not spend $14 million to study anything unless they have a strong suspicion that the compounds work. Based on all of the currently available data, the compounds are, in fact, effective. Many patients are already telling me this, and I really can't see waiting until 2005 to get the results of this one study before benefiting from them. (I am a hiker and runner, and I have started using these various substances myself because I want all of the joint protection I can get.)

In regenerating cartilage, there is stirring excitement about a new formulation of vitamin C (specifically calcium ascorbate containing *threonate*). It is the threonate compound combined with the ascorbate that has a powerful role in regenerating cartilage. It is an ideal form of vitamin C to take for joints because it does three important things: It is rapidly absorbed, it stays in the joint tissues longer, and it is excreted slowly. The role of vitamin C in joint health has been documented for many years, but this newly compounded form of vitamin C is particularly useful in joint health.

REVIEWING GOD'S 3–2–3 PLAN

So, you see, there is something you can do about arthritis—to deal with the pain, to decrease inflammation, and to actually restore cartilage. Three of the very best natural pain-fighting substances God has given us are *curcuma,* from the turmeric root; *prunus cerasus,* extracts from tart cherries; and *holy basil,* an ancient herb from India.

The two substances we talked about to decrease inflammation in the joints are *boswellin,* from the gum resin known in Bible times as frankincense, and a powder made from *sea cucumber,* or *Beche-de-Mer,* a marine animal valued for the treatment of arthritis for centuries in China.

However, the three newly proven substances that stop the loss of cartilage in joints and actually help restore it are the really exciting part of the plan. Of course, God has known about them all the time, since He created them for our benefit. Nevertheless, we have entered a new era for the treatment of arthritis, with the growing use of *glucosamine,* derived from the shells of certain deep-sea animals; a new form of *chondroitin,* with a lower molecular weight that the body can absorb more easily; and a new formulation of *vitamin C,* specifically calcium ascorbate containing threonate.

Using the natural substances God has given us, combined with the power of prayer, are the most potent weapons we have for combating major degenerative diseases like arthritis. In coming chapters I also want to talk with you about the vital importance of the *foods* you choose to eat. Remember, God didn't let the first chapter of the Bible end before He started talking about diet, and it's even more important today. Then, *exercise* can and should play an important role in your victory over arthritis—I want to get you on your feet and moving again! There are also several other compounds available in *supplement* form that you should know about and consider making a part of your daily program. And, last but not least, I want to teach you how to *pray for healing of arthritis*.

God has a personal, unique pathway to healing your arthritis. Are you ready to take the next step?

Chapter 2

THE DIETARY
CONNECTION

Chapter 2

THE DIETARY CONNECTION

After years of studying the human body from the standpoint of finding ways to avoid sickness and prevent disease, I am convinced that our choice of foods—what we eat and what we avoid—is the most potent program for good health within our control. Further, I believe the dietary laws of the Bible offer solid guidance and valuable suggestions for people suffering from arthritis.

As if to stress the priority and importance of a proper diet, the very first chapter of the

Bible includes a specific description of what we should eat. It's not complex or difficult at all: "I give you every seed-bearing plant on the face of the whole earth and every tree that has fruit with seed in it. They will be yours for food" (Genesis 1:29 NIV).

A few chapters later this vegetarian regimen was modified to include the flesh of some animals: "Everything that lives and moves will be food for you. Just as I gave you the green plants, I now give you everything" (Genesis 9:3 NIV).

Basically, God's health plan includes eating fruits, vegetables, seeds, grains, and small amounts of animal substances.

God's health plan also includes a couple of "thou shalt not's": don't *eat* fat and don't *be* fat. "This is a lasting ordinance for the generations to come . . ." says the law. "You must not eat any fat or any blood" (Leviticus 3:17 NIV). We are also to avoid obesity: "But take heed to yourselves and be on your guard, lest your hearts be overburdened and depressed (weighed down) with the giddiness and headache and nausea of self-indulgence, drunkenness, and worldly worries" (Luke 21:34 AMP).

YOUR HEALTH IS DIRECTLY LINKED TO WHAT YOU EAT

When God entered a healing covenant with His people, He immediately shifted the focus to what they should eat, giving specific instructions as to how they should gather and prepare their food. In Exodus 23:25 God promised to place a blessing on the bread and water (the daily food) of His people. With His blessing, God indicated that He would "take sickness away from the midst of [them]."

The Surgeon General of the United States a few years ago reaffirmed God's nutritional laws by stating, "Your choice of diet can influence your long-term health prospects more than any other action you might take."

Traditional medical thinking has taught doctors that what a person eats really has no effect on the pain and inflammation of arthritis. This teaching is biting the dust because of dramatic new understanding of how diet does affect compounds in our body, which in turn either stimulate or suppress inflammation.

The story is a little complex and involves a lot of biochemistry, but bear with me. I think you will find it interesting and very helpful in protecting your own joints.

Basically, the pain associated with arthritis is really the result of inflammation. Inflammation in the body is mediated or caused by compounds such as *prostaglandins* and *cytokines*. Our diet enables us to provide a balance between the compounds that promote or cause inflammation and those that block inflammation.

From a simple point of view, this means that vegetable oils need to be eliminated from your diet. You need to stop using sunflower, safflower, soy, and corn oils and switch to an anti-inflammatory oil such as extra-virgin olive oil or canola oil.

THE OMEGA-6 VERSUS OMEGA-3 BATTLE

Here's how it works. What you eat determines the number of inflammatory compounds in your body. One of the building blocks for inflammatory compounds (the bad guys) is *linoleic acid,* which is especially concentrated in the vegetable oils we just mentioned—sunflower, safflower, and corn, for example.

Your body converts linoleic acid into what are known as omega–6 fatty acids, which include a really bad guy known as *arachidonic acid.* COX–2 is a chemical compound that converts arachidonic acid to PGE2 (prostaglandin E2) and various cytokines (IL–1, IL–6, and TNFa), which are all bad guys that inflame joints and lead to pain.

God designed the body to balance these bad guys with anti-inflammatory compounds such as *alpha linolenic acid,* which is found in coldwater fish—salmon, cod, herring, and mackerel—as well as in flaxseed and leafy green vegetables. Given an ample supply of these good guys, the body converts alpha linolenic acid to the omega–3 fatty acids, EPA and DHA. These are the same good omega–3 fatty acids that are found also in coldwater fish.

You see, your body has two mechanisms for getting the good omega–3s. It can make them from compounds found in flaxseed, green leafy vegetables, and coldwater fish as well as getting the omega–3s directly from the fish.

Many scientists now feel that we are facing more and more inflammatory disorders (this includes lupus, fibromyalgia, chronic fatigue syndrome, etc.) because of our imbalanced intake of the omega–6 fatty acids versus the omega–3s. In times past, people consumed pretty close to equal amounts of the inflammatory omega–6s (the bad guys) and the anti-inflammatory omega–3 fatty acids (the good guys).

Over the past three to four decades, however, Americans have increasingly consumed more of the omega–6 fatty acids without increasing their intake of omega–3s. Some experts estimate that we are now eating ten to twenty times more omega–6s than we are omega–3s. This sets the stage for a powerful, chronic, ongoing inflammatory reaction in the body.

Inflammation is now implicated in heart disease, Alzheimer's disease, and stroke, as well as arthritis. Some scientists at the University of California at Berkeley estimate that chronic inflammation and infection contribute to nearly one-third of all cancers.

NATURAL TOOLS TO FIGHT INFLAMMATION

Recent studies further indicate that corn oil (high in omega–6s) increases COX–2 activity, which leads to an increase in the highly inflammatory prostaglandins. On the other hand, fish oil, which is abundant in the omega–3s, counteracts the COX–2 activities.[1] That is, it inhibits COX–2 activity, which is the way Vioxx, Celebrex, and other medical compounds work to stop inflammation.

Research over the past few years has also shown that these inflammatory omega–6 fatty acids increase colon cancer, whereas the omega–3 fatty acids *prevent* colon cancer. This goes along with the same evidence we have discovered independently related to the COX–2 inhibitors.

If you take the traditional American diet, which has way too many omega–6 fatty acids, and combine it with too little vitamin E, you really make things worse in a hurry, because the inflammatory cytokine IL–1, mentioned earlier, triggers the release of more and more free radicals. (Free radicals are atoms formed when oxygen interacts with certain molecules. These highly reactive radicals can start a chain reaction that damages important cellular components, such as DNA or the cell membrane, causing impaired function or death of the cell.)

If you are low in vitamin E and other antioxidants (the body's defense system against free radicals), a vicious destructive cycle is set up in your body. Few people are getting adequate antioxidant protection in their diet—you need a minimum of seven daily servings of vegetables and fruits. In America, people who eat that many servings are pretty rare.

So how do we get this ratio back into proper balance? We have to reduce prostaglandin and cytokine levels by exchanging vegetable oils for olive oil. In basic terms, get off of the processed foods and get simple. Start eating healthier meals, such as a simple tossed salad with olive oil, some steamed vegetables, and baked chicken, and you will be well on your way to restoring the balance between the omega–6s and the omega–3s.

This imbalance, however, exists deep within your body cells, and supplements are the quickest way (in addition to a healthy diet, of course) to restore this balance. For all my patients, I recommend immediately adding a daily supplement to decrease inflammation in the body and restore the omega–6 balance.

(We will discuss the supplements you should consider in chapter 3.)

After the rather technical and involved explanation of the inflammation-producing omega–6 fatty acids, which are definitely linked to the alarming increase of arthritis in America today, I want to broaden our discussion to cover what I believe is the most beneficial diet, or eating plan, available. While I recommend it for everyone, it is especially important for arthritis sufferers. I also want to deal with some specific foods that are of special interest and concern to people with arthritis.

A DIETARY LIFESTYLE FOR BETTER HEALTH

A great intrigue has arisen in medical and health circles today about the foods that have been eaten for centuries in the lands of the Bible. The diet of Middle Eastern people is of particular interest. One name given to this group of foods that both prevent and help to cure diseases is the Mediterranean diet.

Key characteristics of this dietary lifestyle include:

An abundance of plant foods, including fruits, vegetables, whole grains, beans, nuts, and seeds, either eaten raw or with minimal processing.

A relatively high intake of monounsaturated fat in the form of olive oil. Current research has established that olive oil is a good source of antioxidants and is essentially neutral with respect to the effects of serum cholesterol—in fact, it may actually increase HDL (good) cholesterol.

Low to moderate consumption of dairy prod-

ucts, primarily cheese and yogurt, with little use of fresh milk. The live bacterial cultures of yogurt certainly contribute to the overall healthiness of the diet.

Sparing use of fish, poultry, and red meat. All foods from animal sources are used sparingly, either to flavor other dishes or as a main course on special occasions. Traditionally, the total red meat and poultry consumed was about fifteen ounces per week, with another five to fifteen ounces of fish.

The Mediterranean diet also includes dark, chewy, crusty bread along with pasta, rice, wheat in the form of couscous, bulgur, and potatoes. Notice that this diet is very similar to the one described in Genesis that God prescribed for the first people on earth.

My wife, Linda, and I personally use a variation of the Mediterranean diet for our daily menu. I also recommend it to my patients as one of the best-balanced and most beneficial eating plans available. "Today, it has been scientifically proved that the traditional Mediterranean food is healthy," according to a report from a French health agency. "Even nutritionists praise the Mediterranean diet as a healthy way of eating."

As a Christian believer and a medical doctor, I am convinced that modern people can derive much benefit from the health laws and the moral directives of the Bible. Every single thing we are discovering in science today parallels and bolsters what the Bible says about nutrition. Science is truly "walking in the footsteps of God."

When I was in premed, I was astonished that the dietary laws given in the ancient biblical texts revealed truths that scientists were only beginning to uncover in my day. After decades of intensive personal research, I believe more than ever that even with the amazing medical advances of our times, science is still in the position of "catching up" with the ancient laws God gave His people millennia ago in the Bible. They are still for us today.

Now let's take a quick look at some particular foods that have special significance to you if you are living with arthritis.

THE GARLIC/ONION CONNECTION WITH ARTHRITIS

Increased consumption of garlic and onions has definitely been shown to have a beneficial effect on the symptoms of arthritis. One study that was primarily looking at garlic in connection to heart disease also found that garlic eaters were getting a marked decrease in joint pain, especially the pain associated with degenerative osteoarthritis.

The reason for this became clear to the researchers. Garlic inhibits one of the inflammation-causing prostaglandin hormones.

Onions are a cousin of garlic, but they also contain a moderate amount of sulfur, which is critical for the rebuilding of cartilage, bone, and the various ligaments around the joints. These two foods are always good additions to your diet.

MILK AND ARTHRITIS

Can milk be a contributor to arthritis symptoms? Studies indicate that it certainly may be a factor. Researchers have found that patients suffering from the typical symptoms of both osteoarthritis and rheumatoid arthritis have had a marked reduction in pain and swelling when they've eliminated milk from their diet.

In many of these cases it was discovered that the patients were deficient in the enzyme, lactase, that breaks down the milk sugar, lactose. The other theory connecting milk and arthritis seems even more plausible to me.

The protein found in cow's milk may actually trigger an overreaction of the body's immune system, leading to inflammation. This is an important process in rheumatoid arthritis, an autoimmune disease in which the joint lining swells, invading surrounding tissues and producing chemical substances that attack and destroy the joint surface.[2] We have also seen some indication that milk consumption may be a factor in Type–1 diabetes, an immune-system disease.

Many people with common upper-respiratory allergies improve when they eliminate milk from their diet, also implying a connection between the large-milk protein and stimulation of the body's immune system.

I suggest that milk consumption be limited (better yet, stopped) if you are experiencing arthritic-related symptoms, particularly those related to rheumatoid arthritis.

WHY CORN MAY BE A NO-NO!

Several studies have implicated corn (and especially corn oil) as a major food contributor to arthritis symptoms. It may be that certain people have allergic reactions to corn that trigger the immune system to produce arthritic symptoms.

In one study done in England, corn topped the list of foods that provoked symptoms of arthritis, and wheat products were close behind.

As I explained earlier in this chapter, corn oil is certainly a factor in contributing to the inflammation of arthritis because of the high content of omega–6 fatty acids, which contain arachidonic acid (which is converted to the "bad guys," prostaglandins and cytokines, that inflame joints and cause pain).

If you are experiencing arthritic symptoms of either osteoarthritis or rheumatoid arthritis, try getting off of all corn products for a week or so to see if you are one of those persons who is sensitive to corn. Regardless of whether or not you are having symptoms, I recommend that you avoid corn oil and its related cousins, sunflower oil, safflower oil, etc.

While an allergy to corn would be specific only to certain individuals, the consumption of corn oil is universally detrimental to all of us, upsetting the omega–6/omega–3 balance. We all need to avoid inflammation in our body as much as possible.

Good alternatives to corn oil are olive oil and cold-pressed canola oil, preferably natural. I know there has been some bad press on the dangers of canola oil, but most of this is fictitious information. Canola oil is perfectly safe and much healthier than the corn oils.

In fact, a recent article on the people of Okinawa—who enjoy the greatest longevity of any people group in the world—reported that they traditionally have used canola oil to stir-fry food. Olive oil, as you probably know, is a staple in the Mediterranean countries. The people there also enjoy long life spans and low-ered risk from several killer diseases.

SHOULD ARTHRITIS SUFFERERS AVOID TOMATOES?

The theory that members of the night-shade family—which includes tomatoes, green peppers, eggplant, and white potatoes—can trigger arthritic symptoms has been around for a long time. It is based on the idea that a chemical found in these foods, known as *solanine,* can contribute to arthritic pain and dis-comfort.

Frankly, the science supporting this theory is sparse. Absolutely no controlled studies demonstrate that these foods are arthritic trig-gers. In fact, most of the studies have indicated a strong beneficial effect in the use of tomatoes, and no ill effects have been found from peppers and eggplants.

I personally do not advocate avoiding tomatoes and their cousins to alleviate arthritis symptoms, as the known benefits of this group of foods seem to be increasing in regard to our overall health.

EAT SARDINES TO STOP ARTHRITIS!

How could sardines be an effective treatment for arthritis? It is related to the high content of the omega–3 fatty acids found in certain coldwater fish. I personally enjoy sardines (the water-packed variety) and eat them often. Linda does not like them and is not particularly fond of my consuming them, either, because of the telltale evidence that tends to linger.

If you are not a sardines fan, go for their cousins (salmon, mackerel, herring, cod, halibut, albacore and bluefin tuna, and trout), all coldwater fish that are high in the beneficial omega–3s. Scientists at Albany Medical College in New York have conducted studies on the benefits of the oil contained in these fish. There are at least half a dozen double-blind studies showing that moderate amounts of fish oil do indeed reduce arthritic symptoms.

The marine fatty acids decrease inflammatory compounds such as *leukotrienes*. When these compounds are reduced, inflammation and joint tenderness are reduced. You do have to stay on the fish oils daily, but there is no question about their anti-inflammatory benefits. I recommend taking fish oil capsules, since it is hard to eat six or seven ounces of salmon or two cans of sardines every day.

Check your labels, but increase your intake of EPA, which is one of the common omega–3 fatty acids, to 1.8 grams daily. However, don't get too much of the omega–3s in capsule form, as they are blood thinners.

I heartily recommend that you consider a wholesome, Bible-based eating plan like the Mediterranean diet. There is an abundance of sources about this in numerous books and on the Internet. (You can also find in-depth information in my books *The Doctor and the Word* and *The Bible Cure*.) This dietary lifestyle, combined with a supplement program to gain other important compounds, can help you overcome arthritis and other inflammatory conditions in your body. God is providing scientists with an incredible outpouring of information in these days.

Chapter 3

GOD'S HEALING PRESCRIPTION: TRANSFORMING YOUR LIFE WITH NATURAL SUPPLEMENTS

Chapter 3

GOD'S HEALING PRESCRIPTION:
TRANSFORMING YOUR LIFE
WITH NATURAL SUPPLEMENTS

More than any generation before us, our body is under constant attack. We face pesticides and herbicides in our food, pollution in each breath, a thinning ozone layer, and other damage inflicted on our body every day.

At creation, God placed on earth all foods necessary to maintain our body, our "earthen vessel." He gave us the vitamins, minerals, herbs, antioxidants, essential fatty acids, plant extracts, and other nutrients our body needs to prevent illness and to maintain, improve, or restore our health as necessary. I believe all these nutrients are part of God's "healing prescription" to help us prosper in health and live an abundant life.

Unfortunately, most people find it increasingly difficult to get and use the foods and herbs that God intended to be part of our daily diet. Either they are not readily available or people have bought into today's "fast food" mentality that provides too much of the wrong things and little, if any, of the essential nutrients God intended our body to use.

I believe this is why there seem to be more people suffering from sickness and disease than ever despite the amazing growth of medical technology and the development of new and more effective pharmaceuticals. In a land of great blessing and material prosperity, something is missing.

Throughout my medical practice, I have specialized not only in the diagnosis of disease but also in the use of nutrition, exercise, and ways to recapture the benefits of substances and compounds God put on earth for our use. I have championed the use of natural supplements that are concentrations of those original foods.

WHY I BELIEVE IN SUPPLEMENTS

I firmly believe that in this day and age we should seek quality nutritional supplements to get the vitamins, minerals, antioxidants, and other nutrients we need for optimal health. It's hard to argue with science—medical studies consistently show that people do better when taking nutritional supplements. One recent study found that supplementing with only moderate amounts of nutrients improved mental performance in seniors and enhanced their resistance to disease (*Nutrition,* September, 2001).

Another study suggested that the use of only three supplements—vitamin E, folic acid, and zinc—could save $20 billion in annual hospital costs in the United States by reducing health problems associated with nutritional deficiencies (*Western Journal of Medicine,* May, 1997).

There was a time when most people believed that if they ate a reasonable, well-balanced diet, they got all the vitamins and minerals their body needed. Unfortunately, this is not true today. I think everyone should take, at a minimum, a good multipurpose vitamin each day. There are other minerals and nutrients we need that are also available in supplement form.

For example, if you are fighting arthritis, you will need specific compounds we've talked about—like curcumin, boswellin, glucosamine, and chondroitin. I also recommend taking tart-cherry-fruit powder, holy-basil-leaf extract, sea cucumber, and extra vitamin C (in calcium ascorbate form). These are the absolute basics, the minimum supplements every arthritic patient should be taking.

Obviously, there are other compounds in supplement form that I believe to be very helpful. Let's look at just a few of them.

OMEGA-3 ESSENTIAL FATTY ACIDS

The omega-3s, EPA and DHA, are found in fish oil. They help stop COX-2 and block the highly inflammatory cytokines while promoting the good anti-inflammatory, prostaglandin E1. You should take 600 mg. of EPA/DHA daily.

GAMMA LINOLENIC ACID

Though technically an omega–6 fatty acid, gamma linolenic acid (GLA) is highly anti-inflammatory. GLA, like omega–3s, increases the good prostaglandin E1 and can dramatically decrease arthritic symptoms when taken daily.

All of us need this important compound whether or not we are having symptoms, simply to keep inflammation levels low in our body. I recommend taking cold-pressed evening primrose oil, containing 90 mg. of GLA, every day.

TOCOPHEROLS AND TOCOTRIENOLS

We used to simply recommend that people take vitamin E, but we now have more enlightenment on the whole family of vitamin-E compounds. Natural D-alpha tocopherol is the form of vitamin E we should take daily at a dose of 800 IU. This form of vitamin E counters the effects of COX–2 and prostaglandin E2, which promote inflammation.

The natural D-alpha form should not be taken alone but combined with natural mixed tocopherols as well as a less familiar compound known as tocotrienols. In nature, the tocotrienols (which are cousins of vitamin E) always occur together, and they work best when taken together in a supplement.

One study found that arthritis patients taking supplements of natural vitamin E for four months had a 50 percent reduction in joint pain.[1]

VITAMIN C

Vitamin C will always be on the list of anti-inflammatory compounds our body needs. Vitamin C not only counters inflammation but it also protects cells from the free-radical damage caused by inflammation. Everyone should take vitamin C in the form of ascorbic acid and calcium ascorbate.

If you are fighting arthritis, you should add vitamin C with threonate, which is especially helpful for arthritic cartilage changes. Vitamin C should be taken at a minimum dose of 2,000 mg. daily.

POLYPHENOLS AND FLAVONOIDS

I currently recommend that patients take polyphenols daily because of their anti-inflammatory effect that inhibits the COX–2 enzyme. Green tea is an excellent source of these polyphenols. Another important compound is quercetin, which blocks inflammation.

All of these work extremely well when combined with grape-seed and grape-skin extracts. Be sure that a general bioflavonoid complex is taken, which includes various chemicals such as Hesperidin, Naringin, and others.

OTHER IMPORTANT SUBSTANCES

Other important substances typically found in the better daily supplements that are beneficial for joint health include boron, zinc, magnesium, copper, manganese, and silica.

Another interesting compound proven to combat inflammation is bromelain, which is derived from the stem and stalk of the pineapple. Use of this substance has been found to reduce inflammation up to 60 percent by attacking prostaglandin E2.

There are other herbs that may be useful to patients with arthritis, although they have not yet been studied as extensively as those mentioned above. Herbs such as celery, feverfew, willow yucca, and devil's claw have all produced certain degrees of relief in various patients, though they are not always consistent in their results.

I have been asked on occasion about other arthritic treatment supplements such as SAM-e and MSM. There is, in fact, some promise for SAM-e, but current data indicates that it primarily relieves pain and does not perform a restorative function to the cartilage. A major deterrent to its widespread use is its extremely high cost. Evidence indicates that other less expensive compounds can relieve pain and inflammation equally as well.

I've also received questions about MSM (methyl sulfonyl methane) being marketed as a safe, effective arthritis therapy. Though generally considered to be safe, it is a cousin to DMSO, which is a byproduct of wood processing that has been linked to skin irritation and vision impairment. MSM's pain-relieving function is probably not as effective as compounds like curcumin and other natural COX–2 inhibitors.

WHERE CAN YOU GET THESE SUPPLEMENTS?

All of the vitamins, minerals, and nutritive compounds I've mentioned are generally available at most good vitamin and health-food stores. While there are often scores of choices for each compound, be sure to check labels to compare the quantity and strength of the active ingredients. Also be aware of the potency, purity, and quality of the product, as well as price.

For the past few years I have been working with a group of researchers to research, formulate, and manufacture a line of *Pathway to Healing* products especially designed for specific health concerns. In addition to a basic, multi-purpose daily natural supplement foundation, I have a formulation that combines the eight most potent supplements proven to help prevent and heal arthritis symptoms. It's called Joint Support and is available only from the manufacturer, Natural Alternatives, at (800) 339-5952.

For online information, visit *www.AbundantNutrition.com.*

Chapter 4

GETTING BACK
ON YOUR FEET

Chapter 4

GETTING BACK ON YOUR FEET

As we have seen, you can help your body fight disease or you can bring destruction to your body by what you put in your mouth. Likewise, the exercise you get—or fail to get—also affects your body, the temple of the Holy Spirit.

People protest all the time, "But, Dr. Cherry, it doesn't say in the Bible to exercise." Jesus didn't say much about exercise because the people in His day had no choice but to get plenty of it. They walked every place they went, sometimes twenty or thirty miles at a time. Jesus and His disciples walked from Galilee to Jerusalem and around Judea and Samaria.

There were no "labor-saving conveniences" in those days. People did a great deal of lifting, carrying, pushing, climbing, and other physical labor just doing the necessary daily chores— tending animals, getting water, preparing food. Life was more strenuous no matter what your occupation.

Today some people have a hard time working exercise into their daily routine. Nevertheless, a sensible, regular program of exercise is essential to maintain your body in good condition.

My wife, Linda, a nurse, understands the importance of both good nutrition and adequate exercise for wholeness and health—however, she doesn't enjoy exercise to the degree that I do. I am a runner and like to run four to five miles several days a week when my schedule permits.

Linda exercises, too—she just goes about it differently. She hates to perspire but has adjusted to it in order to get an adequate workout. Much of the time she exercises indoors on a NordicTrack skiing simulator, which provides great exercise for the arms, upper body, and legs, as well as the heart and lungs.

FIND WHAT WORKS FOR YOU

Running may be too strenuous or difficult for some people, so I've encouraged many patients to walk instead. This may be good advice for you as well. You may even have to start slow and work your way up, with a goal of eventually walking up to three miles in forty to forty-five minutes, three to five times a week.

Your body needs forty-five minutes of exercise at least three days a week—enough to get your heart rate up. And you don't need expensive gym equipment or a membership in a health club to do it. Just walking the dog every day might be a good way to start. Or you could go to the mall and walk from one end to the other and back again. Just keep moving—don't turn your head and look in the stores. Save that for later.

There are a lot of myths about exercise. One of them is that arthritis is caused by too much exercise. Just the opposite is true. The worst thing you can do is to be sedentary. Runners who go jogging or running for miles at a time have less arthritis than people who sit around.

While injury and trauma can increase arthritis, weight-bearing exercise may actually prevent it. This seems to be a contradictory statement, but low-impact exercise apparently places just the right amount of tension on the joint pad to cause the diffusion of nourishing and protective chemicals into the cartilage.

Exercise can aggravate existing arthritis, but if you are not suffering arthritic pain, weight-bearing exercise can be very useful. Studies consistently show that cartilage likes to be used, and physical activity will actually stimulate cartilage growth and repair.

Exercise helps relieve and prevent the problems associated with arthritis, such as joint stiffness, muscle weakness, joint deformity, and depression. Three types of exercise are best for people with arthritis:

Range-of-motion exercises help maintain normal joint movement and relieve stiffness. They also help maintain or increase flexibility.

Strengthening exercises help keep or increase muscle strength. Strong muscles help support and protect joints affected by arthritis. Weight-bearing exercise can help minimize the effects of osteoarthritis.

Aerobic or *endurance* exercises improve cardiovascular fitness, help control weight, and improve overall function. Aerobic exercise can reduce inflammation in some joints. Weight control can be important to people who have arthritis because extra weight puts extra pressure on many joints. In fact, being overweight and out of shape can set the stage for developing arthritis. As a rule of thumb, men should have only about 15 percent body fat and women about 22 percent. Exercise can play an important role in any successful weight-reduction plan.

DETERMINE YOUR SAFE HEART-RATE RANGE

Whatever exercise you choose, work at it vigorously enough to get your heart rate elevated during the time you are exercising. Physical fitness experts have a simple formula for determining a safe heart-rate range for exercising. Simply subtract your age from 220 to find your maximum heart rate. Say you're age forty: Your formula would be 220 − 40 = 180.

Your target heart-rate zone is between 60 and 80 percent of that number. So multiply your maximum heart rate by 60 percent for the bottom of your safe exercise range and by 80 percent for the top. As you exercise, check your pulse rate now and then, and be sure your heartbeat is within that range.

Find your pulse in your wrist or neck, count the number of beats in ten seconds, and multiply that number by six. If the number you get is within your safe exercise range, you're fine. If it's lower, work harder. If it's higher, slow down a little.

When starting an exercise program, aim at the lowest part of your target zone for the first few weeks. Gradually build up to the higher part of your target zone.

IT'S NEVER TOO LATE

I've heard people say, "Well, it's too late now. I hurt too bad to exercise—I can hardly walk. The cartilage in my knees is already degenerated—or my hips hurt when I try to move. Exercising is only going to make it worse."

Wrong. Exercise can be very beneficial to the person with arthritis. When you're sedentary, the fluids in the joints don't have a chance to mix, to flux, to move in and out of the cartilage. Exercise is kind of like the agitator in a washing machine. The agitator keeps things stirred up. The constant motion squeezes the various fluids in the joints in and out and makes the cartilage more elastic and thicker with more of a cushioning effect.

As I said, I prefer walking or running—my wife, Linda, prefers walking or using the NordicTrack. Swimming is another good exercise that is easy on the weight-bearing joints. Any exercise that causes a constant motion in the joints helps stir the fluids in the cartilage that keeps it supple and flexible, so it won't collapse and degenerate.

Maybe you're a person who hasn't taken very good care of your "temple," your body. Well, it's never too late to start. Even if you've worn out the cartilage in your knee joints, and weight-bearing exercises are painful, you can use a stationary cycle or go to water exercises.

USE IT OR LOSE IT

It's really true! Not using any part of your body for a long period of time will make it weak or cause it to lose its function. For example, if you put your arm in a sling for several weeks, it would begin to atrophy, getting smaller and weaker. People who are bedridden for any length of time get progressively weaker.

That's why exercising all our body's systems regularly is so vitally important.

In our lean-back-and-relax, remote-control society, people want everything to be easy, but your body needs regular exercise. If you haven't been getting any kind of physical workout, exercising may be hard at first, but the more you do it, the more your body will respond. You can't just go to the store and buy some pills, go home and take them, and then sit on the couch eating potato chips and watching TV. You've got to get up and move. Take an activity break and do your exercise!

Walking, jogging, stationary cycling, outdoor cycling, water exercise, and swimming are all fine workouts. The important thing is to find something you can do regularly that exercises the skeletal system and builds the aerobic capacity of your heart and lungs.

Combine various kinds of exercise—aerobics promote fitness, loosen muscles and joints, and strengthen the heart and lungs. Weightlifting increases strength, builds up muscle mass, strengthens the tendons, and stabilizes the joints better.

Stretching exercises are also important. They strengthen the ligaments that support the joints and make them more supple. Exercise tightens the ligaments and tendons, while stretching loosens them. So take time to stretch after each exercise session. Over time, it will give you a greater range of motion.

Exercise, like nutrition, must be balanced. Your goal is to be flexible, aerobically fit, and strong. You must begin your exercise program and increase exercise time and intensity gradually—a crash exercise program is no better than a crash diet.

Be safe—avoid injury. Be cautious—avoid overstrain. Be dedicated—do it daily. You'll find yourself feeling better physically, emotionally, and mentally, with a rejuvenating sense of well-being.

Chapter 5

PRAYING WITH UNDERSTANDING

Chapter 5

PRAYING WITH UNDERSTANDING

"I will pray with the spirit, and I will pray with the understanding also" (1 Corinthians 14:15 KJV).

I believe you should pray and ask God for the healing of your arthritis. Now that you know more about the disease and how it is attacking your body, you are better equipped to pray with understanding and expect your prayer to be answered. This is an absolutely vital part of finding and following your pathway to healing.

God has invited us to pray about all our needs, anything that concerns us. He has given us faith to believe for answers to our prayers. He has made it abundantly clear that it is His will to heal us, and He has promised that our praying will get results. Jesus said, "Ask, and it shall be given you; seek, and ye shall find; knock, and it shall be opened unto you: for every one that asketh receiveth; and he that seeketh findeth; and to him that knocketh it shall be opened" (Matthew 7:7–8).

So what are we waiting for? Prayer should be our first recourse, not our last resort!

Sometimes people ask, "Why should I have to ask God for things if He is all-knowing and already is aware of my needs?" Quaker theologian Richard Foster answers that question by saying simply:

God likes to be asked. We like our

children to ask us for things that we already know they need because the very asking enhances and deepens the relationship. P. T. Forsyth notes, "Love loves to be told what it already knows. . . . It wants to be asked for what it longs to give."[1]

Prayer releases our anointing or power to take our spiritual authority over disease.

SPEAKING TO THE MOUNTAIN

How do we pray for healing? Specifically rather than generally. For example, if I were sick and you were going to pray for me, I wouldn't want you to say, "Oh, God, please heal everybody who is sick today." The problem would not be that I didn't want other sick people to get well but rather that I need a strong, directed prayer that releases healing power to overcome my particular attack.

I need a specific, faith-filled prayer to overcome my problem and restore my body. This is what I call "speaking to the mountain of disease" when you pray.

Jesus said, "If anyone says to this mountain, 'Go, throw yourself into the sea,' and does not doubt in his heart but believes that what he says will happen, it will be done for him" (Mark 11:23 NIV).

So I believe that when we pray for healing we should speak to the specific mountain of sickness and command it to be gone. We have this authority as believers.

So many times I have seen what medicine calls "spontaneous remission" (I call it a healing by the power of God) occur when a patient speaks to a specific mountain of disease. As we seek and follow God's pathway, we see healing that cannot be explained by medical science.

When you pray, be bold and assertive. Don't be apologetic or timid. Be as aggressive in your praying as you are in seeking medical information. Martin Luther, the great Protestant reformer, described how he prayed for his sick friend, Melanchthon, also a leader of the church:

> I besought the Almighty with great vigor . . . quoting from Scripture all the promises I could remember, that prayers should be granted, and said that he must grant my prayer, if I was henceforth to put faith in his promises.[2]

YOUR PRAYER DOESN'T BOTHER GOD

Remember that you are not bothering God with your requests when you pray. Nothing is too great or too small to bring to Him. After all, He invites you to come to Him with your needs and cast your cares upon Him. The *Amplified Bible*'s version of 1 Peter 5:7 says, "Casting the whole of your care [all your anxieties, all your worries, all your concerns, once and for all] on Him, for He cares for you affectionately and cares about you watchfully."

For more than fifty years Oral Roberts has been known as a man of faith and prayer. He was a pioneer in seeking to merge the healing streams of prayer and medicine, personally praying for multiplied thousands of sick people over time. He also built a large hospital complex in Tulsa, Oklahoma, called the City of Faith, which was operated by Christian doctors, nurses, and staff who prayed with the patients as well as treated them medically. He was years ahead of his time. What was regarded as a bit radical then is now being studied, taught, and practiced by physicians and institutions across the country.

Brother Roberts says that the best way to be sure your prayer is answered . . . is to pray!

God challenges you to do unlimited asking. To the one in need of salvation, He says, "Him that cometh to me I will in no wise cast out" (John 6:37). To the one in need of healing, He says, "I will come and heal him" (Matthew 8:7). To the one tormented by fear or dogged by failure, He says, "Come unto me . . . and I will give you rest" (Matthew 11:28). To the one who is a slave to habit, He says, "If the Son therefore shall make you free, ye shall be free indeed" (John 8:36).

Are you expecting an answer? If you

expect the Lord to do wonderful things for you, He will. Believe it, and you will find, as I have, that prayer is one of the most wonderful experiences ever known.[3]

LET'S PRAY RIGHT NOW

Are you ready to pray for God's healing touch in your body? With all my heart I believe He wants to heal you. It may be that your recovery will come quickly, even supernaturally, as He sends His Word to heal you. Perhaps He will use your doctor and medical care to take away the pain and restore the damage to your joints. Or He may use the natural substances He created in supplement form to fight the inflammation and restore the cartilage. Maybe He will use a combination of all three healing streams to make you whole.

But now it is time to ask Him for healing . . . and to believe. I have provided a detailed, specific prayer for you to use. Pray it often, until the words and the details are second nature to you. Pray, and keep on praying. Ask, and keep on asking. Believe, and keep on believing.

A Prayer for Healing From Arthritis

Father, I come before you in the name of your precious Son, Jesus, thanking you that Jesus bore in His own body two thousand years ago the symptoms of the infirmity of arthritis. I thank you that because He bore this disease in His own body, I was healed!

Therefore, Father, I am coming before you, seeking the manifestation of that healing in my physical body. In the name of Jesus, I speak to the cartilage in my joints [name the joint where you are suffering pain, i.e., knee, hip, ankle, shoulder, etc.], and I command that cartilage to increase in thickness and become more pliable and more elastic.

I further pray that the inflammatory cells that lead to swelling and pain will be removed from that joint. I say in Jesus' name that I will be able to move that joint and serve you day to day without pain, symptom, or inflammation in my body.

Father, as I do all I can do in the natural, I look to you to do the supernatural that I cannot do. I send forth the healing, anointing power of the Holy Spirit, the Comforter, who resides within me, to come into my body and into my joints, and I speak comfort and healing to these joints.

Thank you, Father, that the manifestation of my healing is on the way. I praise you, Father, *that you are revealing the specific pathway that I need to walk in that will lead to my healing. I thank you for all of these things in the precious name of Jesus, and I close this prayer praising you and thanking you because through my eyes of faith, I see myself healing. In Jesus' name. Amen.*

YOUR NEXT STEPS IN GOD'S PATHWAY TO HEALING

You have begun an important journey in finding your pathway to healing arthritis by reading this book and beginning to act upon the truths you have received.

Let's review and summarize the steps you need to take now as you receive God's unique pathway to healing for you.

Step 1: See your doctor. Consult a Christian physician or a competent medical doctor. I encourage you to find a Christian doctor who will pray with you and give you all the facts known about your symptoms of arthritis.

Step 2: Pray with understanding. Get as much information as possible about your situation. Review what you have learned in this book. Get current information about your symptoms and condition. Seek God in prayer and ask Him to reveal to you and to your doctor the best steps in the natural you can take in your pathway to healing.

Step 3: Ask the Holy Spirit to guide you to the truth. For example, your doctor may advise you to use a COX–2 inhibitor like Vioxx or Celebrex to combat the pain and inflammation in your joints. He or she may recommend that you make some changes in your daily diet or in your exercise routine. Or he or she may suggest that you begin taking a supplement containing glucosamine and chondroitin. Explore all the aspects of the pathway we have shared with you, the pathway God has created to strengthen and guard your health. Allow the Holy Spirit to guide you to all truth.

Step 4: Maintain proper and healthy nutrition. Exercise and stay fit. We encourage you to stay on the Mediterranean diet and to use the foods, herbs, and supplements we discussed earlier to help your body overcome any painful symptoms of arthritis. Work out a regular program of physical exercise to strengthen your body and to promote flexibility and fitness.

Step 5: Stand firm in God's pathway to healing for you. Refuse to be discouraged or defeated. Keep on keeping on. Be aggressive in prayer and in faith, claiming your healing in Jesus Christ.

We are praying that God will both reveal His pathway to healing arthritis to you and give you the strength and faith to walk in it.

ENDNOTES

Introduction

1. Edward H. Yelin, Ph.D., Professor (Adjunct) of Medicine and Health Policy, University of California, San Francisco, HealingWithNutrition.com http://www.healingwithnutrition.com/adisease/arthritis/arthritis.html.

Chapter 1

1. "MSU study: Tart cherries a painkiller," MedServ Medical News. http://www.medserv.dk/health/1999/02/02/story10.htm.
2. "Sea Cucumber," Nutrition Dynamics, Inc., Health News http://www.nutritiondynamics.com/research_articles31.htm.

Chapter 2

1. Jack Challem, "Natural Alternatives to the Super Aspirins," LetsLiveon-Line.com, 44.
2. "Arthritis, Your Orthopaedic Connection," American Academy of Orthopaedic Surgeons. http://orthoinfo.aaos.org/brochure/thr-report.cfm?Thread-2& topcategory\rthritis.

Chapter 3

1. Jack Challem, "Natural Alternatives to the Super Aspirins," 45.

Chapter 5

1. Richard J. Foster, *Prayer: Finding the Heart's True Home* (San Francisco: Harper San Francisco, 1992).
2. Bengt R. Hoffman, *Luther and the Mystics* (Minneapolis: Augsburg, 1976), 196.
3. Oral Roberts, "Oral Roberts Answers Questions About ... PRAYER," 9. In Reginald Cherry, M.D., *Healing Prayer* (Nashville: Thomas Nelson, 1992), 73–76.

REGINALD B. CHERRY, M.D.—A MEDICAL DOCTOR'S TESTIMONY

The first six years of my life were lived in the dusty rural town of Mansfield, in the Ouachita Mountains of western Arkansas. In those childhood years, I had one seemingly impossible dream—to become a doctor!

Through God's grace, I attended and graduated from Baylor University and the University of Texas Medical School. Throughout those years, I felt God tug on my heart a number of times, especially through Billy Graham as I heard him preach on television. But I never surrendered my life to Jesus Christ.

In those early days of practicing medicine, I met Dr. Kenneth Cooper and became trained in the field of preventive medicine. In the mid-seventies I moved to Houston and established a medical practice for preventive medicine. Sadly, at that time money became a driving force in my life.

Nevertheless, God was good to me. He brought into our clinic a nurse who became a Spirit-filled Christian, and she began praying for me. In fact, she had her whole church praying for me!

In my search for fulfillment and meaning in life, I called out to God one night in late November of 1979 and prayed, "Jesus, I give you everything I own. I'm sorry for the life I've lived. I want to live for you the rest of my days. I give you my life." A doctor had been born again. Oh, and by the way, that beautiful nurse,

Linda, who prayed for me and shared Jesus with me is now my wife!

Not only did Jesus transform my life but He also transformed my medical practice. God spoke to me and said, "I want you to establish a Christian clinic. From now on when you practice medicine, you will be *ministering* to patients." I began to pray for patients seeking God's pathway to healing in the supernatural realm as well as in the natural realm.

Over the years we have witnessed how God has miraculously used both supernatural and natural pathways to heal our patients and to demonstrate His marvelous healing and saving power.

I know what God has done in my life, and I know what God has done in the lives of our patients. He can do the same in yours—He has a unique pathway to healing for you! He is the Lord that heals you (see Exodus 15:26), and by His stripes you were healed (see Isaiah 53:5).

Know that Linda and I are standing with you as you seek God's pathway to healing for joint and arthritis problems and as you walk in His pathway to healing for your life.

If you do not know Jesus Christ as your personal Lord and Savior, I invite you to pray this prayer and ask Jesus into your life:

Lord Jesus, I invite you into my life as my Lord and Savior. I repent of my past sins. I ask you to forgive me. Thank you for shedding your blood on the cross to cleanse me from my sin and to heal me. I receive your gift of everlasting life and surrender all to you. Thank you, Jesus, for saving me. Amen.

ABOUT THE AUTHOR

Reginald B. Cherry, M.D., did his premed at Baylor University, graduated from the University of Texas Medical School, and has practiced diagnostic and preventive medicine for more than twenty-five years. His work in medicine has been recognized and honored by the city of Houston and by President George W. Bush when he was the governor of Texas.

Dr. Cherry and his wife, Linda, a clinical nurse who has worked with Dr. Cherry and his patients during the past two-and-a-half decades, now host the popular television program *The Doctor and the Word*, which has a potential viewing audience of 90 million homes weekly.

They also publish a monthly medical newsletter and produce topical audiocassette teachings, minibooks, and booklets. Dr. Cherry is author of the bestselling books *The Doctor and the Word*, *The Bible Cure*, and *Healing Prayer*.

RESOURCES AVAILABLE FROM REGINALD B. CHERRY MINISTRIES, INC.

Prayers That Heal: Faith-Building Prayers When You Need a Miracle

Combining the wisdom of over twenty-five years of medical practice and the revelation of God's Word, Dr. Cherry provides the knowledge you need to pray effectively against diabetes, cancer, heart disease, eye problems, hypoglycemia, and fifteen other common afflictions that try to rob you of your health.

Healing Prayer

A fascinating, in-depth look at a vital link between spiritual and physical healing. Dr. Cherry presents actual case histories of people healed through prayer, plus the latest information on herbs, vitamins, and supplements that promote vibrant health. This is sound information you need to keep you healthy—mind, soul, and body.

God's Pathway to Healing: Prostate Cancer

This minibook is packed with enlightening insights for men who are searching for ways to prevent prostate cancer or who have actually been diagnosed with this disease. Discover how foods, plant-derived natural supplements, and a change in diet can be incorporated into your life to help you find a pathway to healing for prostate disease.

God's Pathway to Healing: Herbs That Heal

Learn the truth about common herbal remedies and discover the possible side effects of each. Discover which herbs can help treat symptoms of insomnia, arthritis, heart problems, asthma, and many other conditions. Read this book and see if herbs are part of God's pathway to healing for you.

God's Pathway to Healing: Menopause

This minibook is full of helpful advice for women who are going through what can be a very stressful time of life. Find out what foods, supplements, and steps can be taken to find a pathway to healing for menopause and perimenopause.

The Bible Cure (now in paperback)

Dr. Cherry presents hidden truths in the Bible taken from ancient dietary health laws, how Jesus anointed with natural substances to heal, and how to activate faith through prayer for health and healing. This book validates scientific medical research by proving God's original health plan.

The Doctor and the Word (now in paperback)

Dr. Cherry introduces how God has a pathway to healing for you. Jesus healed instantaneously and supernaturally, while other healings involved a process. Discover how the manifestation of your healing can come about by seeking His ways.

Dr. Cherry's *Study Guides, Volume 2* (bound volume)

Receive thirty valuable resource study guides from topics Dr. Cherry has taught on the Trinity Broadcasting Network (TBN) program *The Doctor and the Word*.

Basic Nutrient Support

Dr. Cherry has developed a daily nutrient supplement that is the simplest to take and yet the most complete supplement available today. Protect your body daily with natural substances that fight cancer, heart disease, and many other problems. Call Natural Alternatives at (800) 339–5952 to place your order. Mention service code "BN30" when ordering. (Or, order through the company's Web site: *www.AbundantNutrition.com*.)

Joint Support

You don't have to struggle with the painful symptoms of joint pain and arthritis. Dr. Cherry has formulated a potent supplement containing the key nutrients and extracts from natural substances. Based on his twenty-five years of medical practice and research, this supplement includes everything he recommends to support joint health. Call Natural Alternatives at (800) 339–5952 to place your order. Mention service code "K261" when ordering. (Or, order through the company's Web site: *www.AbundantNutrition.com.*)

Reginald B. Cherry Ministries, Inc.

P.O. Box 27711

Houston, TX 77227-7711

1-888-DRCHERRY

BECOME A PATHWAY TO HEALING PARTNER

We invite you to become a "pathway partner." We ask you to stand with us in prayer and financial support as we provide new programs, resources, books, minibooks, and a unique, one-of-a-kind monthly newsletter.

Our monthly Pathway to Healing Partner Newsletter sorts through the confusion about health and healing. In it, Dr. Cherry shares sensible, biblical, and medical steps you can take to get well. Every issue points you to your pathway to healing. Writing from a Christian physician's Bible-based point of view, Dr. Cherry talks about nutrition and health, how to pray for specific diseases, updates on the latest medical research, Linda's own recipes for healthy eating, and questions and answers about issues you need to know about.

In addition, we'll provide you with Dr. Cherry and Linda's ministry calendar, broadcast schedule, resources for better living, and special monthly offers.

This newsletter is available to you as you partner with the Cherrys through prayer and monthly financial support to help expand this God-given ministry. Pray today about responding with a monthly contribution of $10 or more. Call or write to the following address to find out how you can receive this valuable information.

Become a pathway partner today by writing:

Reginald B. Cherry Ministries, Inc.

P.O. Box 27711

Houston, TX 77227-7711

Visit our Web site:

www.drcherry.org

1-888-DRCHERRY